Setpoint Diet Cookbook:

Lose weight quickly, with easy and delicious recipes

Table of Contents

Disclaimer:

universal. As befitting its nature, it is presented without assurance regarding its prolonged validity or interim quality.

The publisher and author are not responsible for any specific health or allergy needs that may require medical supervision and are not liable for any damages or negatives consequences from any treatment, action, application or preparation, to any person reading or following the information in this book.

Introduction

Congratulations on downloading " Set Point Diet : fast and free diet to weight loss " and thank you for doing so.

Have you heard about the set point diet? If you haven't, you're in for a treat. The set point diet introduce nutritious-yet-delicious eating strategies that eventually lead to permanent maintenance of a healthy weight for life. You won't gain it back, either! Once you lower your set point weight, you'll burn calories like a naturally thin person. No more calorie counting!!!

But it gets even better than that. The set point diet also treats, cures, or reduces the risk of many serious diseases. Studies show most diseases are caused by nutritional issues, by poor-quality diets that damage the body's ability to function properly.

Obesity is not only a symptom of a poor-quality diet, but it also contributes to — or is the underlying cause of — many diseases. You might even say almost all diseases are linked to an overweight or obese condition in one way or another.

The set point diet addresses the nutritional root of the problem, thereby curing obesity and the illnesses it spawns. It has been scientifically proven effective in more than 13,000 peer-reviewed clinical trials to lower the set point weight, leading to permanent weight loss. This reduces the risk for other diseases.

Chapter 1: understanding Set Point Diet and how it works

The Set Point Diet is a food strategy in the 70s. Recently revived and reworked by health magazines of more superfluous, definitely and without too many sacrifices.

What is the set point diet?

The set point diet is an eating plan that focuses on eating the foods proven to heal hormones, restore beneficial gut bacteria, and heal neurological inflammation to lower the set point weight. This is done by consuming foods as close to their natural states as possible. It emphasizes whole foods while reducing highly processed foods and sugars from the diet.

How it works?

This diet provides that according to their caloric intake a score is assigned to each food by creating tables of foods subdivided according to the points: from 0 to 4 points.

There are also tables that link 100 grams of food with the number of points it provides.

The menu is established based on weight, height and gender of the person who will have, based on these parameters, a minimum number and a maximum number of points to be distributed throughout the day. The weight-to-height ratio is defined as the body mass index and the normal values of this parameter range from 20 to 25. After 25, we are in an obesity condition. You can therefore think of doing a points diet, as this diet promises to lose weight around one kilo a week.

The points diet provides a long and tabulated list of foods, giving each of them a given score. By keeping these data in hand, every person can stimulate their culinary vein and create the menus they prefer. Obviously in the composition of the various dishes you must always have an eye to the cumulative score, which should never exceed the maximum imposed by the diet.

Points Calculations

The rules according to which this diet is based come from the different score that food has and from the need for points of the individual calculated on the basis of weight, height and gender.

women of average height (1.55 - 1.70 m)		men of average height (1.70 - 1.85 m)	
Kg from - to	Points from - to	Kg from - to	Points from - to
Up to 70	18 - 24	Up to 80	22 - 26
71 - 80	20 - 25	81 - 90	24 - 29
81 - 90	22 - 27	91 - 100	26 - 30
91 - 100	24 - 29	100 - 110	28 - 32
Over 100	26 - 30	Over 110	30 - 35

the number of points listed above is to be understood as a meal. The diet has a duration of one or two weeks and the points are also attributed to physical activity.

Chapter 2 : Foods to eat on the Set Point Diet

1. Non-starchy vegetables. This is the most important food group in the set point diet, and it should make up about half of your plate for every meal. A non-starchy vegetable is one that you could potentially eat raw (you don't have to, but you could), so corn and potatoes are not included.

2. Nutrient-dense protein. This is the second most important set point diet food group and it should make up about a third of your plate for every meal. Ideally, you want protein from sources such as humanely raised animals. However, don't think that you have to spend a ton of money just to get good protein; canned tuna is just one example of a high-quality and low-cost protein source.

3. Whole-food fats. Most people know by now that good fat doesn't make us fat, but many folks are still getting a lot of their fats from oils. Dieters people get their good fats from whole foods, such as nuts and seeds.

4. Low-fructose fruits. Some fruits pack more sugar than others. On the set point diet, it's recommended to focus on fruits with the lowest amounts of fructose and the highest amount of nutrients. In other words, say hello to berries and citrus fruits.

You might be wondering where to fit the whole-food fats and low-fructose fruits on your ever-growing plate. The set point dieters take a couple of different approaches here. Some folks use whole-food fats and low-fructose fruits to make tasty sauces for their protein or vegetables. Others prefer to use these ingredients to make set point-friendly desserts — such as cakes made with almond flour — once their meals are complete.

Foods and following points

Foods with 0 points

Fruits	Vegetables and legumes	Drinks
Strawberry – apple – pineapple – orange – raspberry – watermelon – medlar - grapefruit	Tomato – celery – aubergine - onions – cabbage - pumpkin – corn - beans – artichokes – carrots - spinach	Thè - coffee – water - herbal infusions

Foods with 1 point

fruits	10-15 cherries ; 3 slices of pineapple ; a glass of fruit juice ; 4 plums ; 15 grains of grapes ; a banana
drinks	A coke (1 , 5 points) ; a non-alcoholic beer
sauce	Oil ; butter ; mayonnaise
meat	2 slices of turkey ; a ham

fish	4 shrimps ; 100 gr. of mussels
Dairy product	2 slices of emmental ; 2 skimmed yogurt ; 1 glass of skimmed milk
Cereals and Carbs	8 tablespoons of whole grains; 2 whole biscuits; 100 grams of boiled potatoes; 1 slice of toast; 2 rice cakes

Foods with 3 points

Drinks	One glass of wine ; one beer
Legumes	5 tablespoons of cooked vegetables; 5 tablespoons of peas
meat	120 gr of turkey or veal; 150 chicken breast
Fish	natural tuna; 120 grams of cod or prawns
Dairy product	1 jar of fruit yogurt; 40 g of white cheese

Cereal and Carbs	120 gr of rice; 50 gr of bread; 2 tablespoons of muesli; 100 g of pasta with vegetables
else	1 egg; half a bar of chocolate; 1 tablespoon of jam; 2 sweet biscuits

Food with 4 points

Cereals and carbs	Dairy product	meat	fish	else
30 gr of fresh pasta	30 gr of emmental	100 gr of salami	100 gr of fresh tuna	2 balls of ice cream

Chapter 3 : pros and cons

Pros

The benefits of this diet relate to weight loss, as it causes you to lose 1 kilo a week. Moreover, it leaves a lot of freedom in the construction of the menus for which it is not one of those diets in which they must be renounced. It is also a diet suitable for those who follow a vegetarian diet because it can exclude all foods of animal origin at will.

Cons

If on the one hand leaving the subject free to choose food is a benefit to psychology, on the other hand it can hurt your health. In fact some subjects can choose to undertake a diet only protein, which can cause many problems to the kidneys and liver, or to the diet a diet rich in fatty foods, with increased cholesterol and triglycerides.

The risk is that it becomes an unbalanced diet and that no caloric intake is needed.

Moreover, a type of diet like this does not help the person to learn to eat well.

The criticism of this diet stems from the fact that the link between the attributed score and the calories of the food is not very real and this diet tends to prefer a high protein and low carb regime as it associates with lower protein foods than those based on carbohydrates .

Chapter 4 : how to make the Set Point Diet work for you

The goal of the set point diet is for its followers to eat so many non-starchy vegetables, nutrient-dense proteins, whole-food fats, and low-fructose fruits (in that order) that they are too full for processed starches, fats, and sweets. That's why it's important to focus on what to do on the set point diet, as opposed to focusing on what not to do.

There are three underlying causes of chronic weight gain that have nothing to do with willpower, have nothing to do with not trying hard enough, or anything along those lines.

Learning more about these causes — which include inflammation in the brain, a deregulated system in the gut, and an imbalance in hormones — can be really helpful during this time. That's because the way that you think about eating can actually make a huge difference while you're changing your diet.

when we feel guilty or shameful about what we're munching on, these feelings can actually have an impact on our hormones and slow down our weight-loss goals and may even fatten us up more. Who wants that?

So, seeing food as an ally to your weight loss rather than the opposition is really key here. Luckily, the set point diet offers many tasty options of meals you can put together to reach your goals and a new set point weight. For example, you might have a green smoothie with leafy greens, avocado, and protein for breakfast. Or perhaps you might opt for scrambling some eggs with veggies and some meat or fish. Lunch and dinner might include a salad or stir fry with some healthy protein.

Just about everyone can find at least one non-starchy vegetable they enjoy. So, if someone hates broccoli but loves asparagus, perhaps their strategy is simply to add more asparagus to their healthy meals. The same goes for protein. At the end of the day.

Chapter 5 : To whom is adapt?

The Set Point diet is suitable for those people who want to lose weight but who are also healthy.

For those suffering from kidney or liver disease it is not indicated because it is very rich in protein.

It is not suitable even for those who do sports as athletes need a lot of macro and micronutrients well established to be able to withstand muscular effort and is not suitable for pregnant women or the elderly because it is not a balanced diet.

Chapter 6 : weekly menu

Let's see now to give advice on the menus. Here is an example of the three points diet menus based on three main meals and two snacks.

Menu n° 1

This menu is calibrated for a woman who weighs less than 70 pounds and has an average height and provides about 22 points.

breakfast	200 ml of partially skimmed milk and 80 gr of cake with jam.
snack	a low-fat yogurt and a kiwi
lunch	50 gr of pasta, 60 gr of bresaola, a teaspoon of oil, peppers.

snack	an apple of about 150 gr
dinner	50 gr of bread, 60 gr of smoked salmon, zucchini, a teaspoon of oil

Menu n° 2

This is a typical 350 point menu and provides about 1260 kcal.

breakfast	a glass of skim milk, three toasted slices to which to add a spoon of jam or honey, a coffee without sugar.
snack	1 apple or an orange juice
lunch	a portion of pasta of about 50 gr to be seasoned with zucchini or with tomato to add a little parmesan, about a teaspoon

snack	a low-fat yogurt or a fruit-based one
dinner	a margherita pizza and a beer or boiled cod with salad dressing to be dressed with oil. Add a portion of bread and a fruit of about 200 gr (example: a banana)

Menu n° 3

This menu provides 18 points and is specific for those who are overweight.

breakfast	choice between: -slice of toast with cheese and eggs, a pear and an orange -a salmon toast, a tangerine or kiwi, a sandwich with turkey and fruit
snack	///

lunch	choice between: tagliatelle with mushrooms, potatoes au gratin with cheese, veal stew
snack	choice between: -milk and biscuits - cappuccino with chocolate - cherry and banana cocktails
dinner	choice between: -chicken salad with cheese -ham and vegetables -a mozzarella and a sandwich -pepperoni

Chapter 7: 0 Points recipes

0 point texas caviar

15 minute prep

Ingredients

1   (14-ounce) can black-eyed peas, rinsed and drained

1/2   cup red bell pepper, chopped

1/2   cup thinly sliced green onions

1/2   cup refrigerated fresh salsa

1/2   cup fresh cilantro, chopped

1   garlic clove, minced

1   tablespoon fresh lime juice

1   teaspoon dried oregano

Directions

Combine all ingredients in a medium bowl; stir until well blended. Cover and chill at least 2 hours or up to 8 hours.

Good served with light tortilla scoops or red bell pepper wedges.

0 point Cucumber Salad

In a large measuring cup mix:

1/4 c. white vinegar

1 TBS lemon juice

2 tsp. liquid sweetener (Agave In The Raw)

1 tsp. salt

1/8 tsp. pepper

1/2 tsp. celery seed

Stir together and pour over sliced cucumber and onion.

In a med/large mixing bowl slice cucumber and onion:

1/2 of a medium sweet onion, sliced (I cut the slices in half and separated the rings)

3-4 medium cucumbers sliced (I used organic).

0 point salsa

Ingredients

1 15 oz can of corn

1 15 oz can of black beans

3-4 Roma Tomatoes, diced

1 jalapeños

1/2 cup red onion

1/2 cup cilantro

Lime

Salt and Pepper to taste

Instructions

Rinse and drain corn and black beans. Add to a medium bowl. Cut or dice the cilantro, onion, jalapeno, tomatoes and add them to the bowl. Squeeze in some lime juice and add salt and pepper. Enjoy with chips!

0 point beet chips

1/2 of recipe (about 1 cup): 97 calories, 0.5g total fat (0g sat fat), 466mg sodium, 21.5g carbs, 6.5g fiber, 15g sugars, 3.5g protein

Prep: 10 minutes

Cook: 2 1/2 hours

Ingredients:

1 lb. (2 - 4) raw beets

1/4 tsp. salt

Directions:

Preheat oven to 250 degrees. Spray two baking sheets with olive oil nonstick spray.

Using a mandoline slicer, cut beets into 1/8-inch-thick rounds.

Lay beet rounds on the sheets, evenly spaced.

Lightly mist with olive oil nonstick spray, and sprinkle with salt.

Bake for 1 hour and 15 minutes.

Carefully remove the baking sheets, and return them to the oven on the opposite racks. (No need to flip the chips.)

Bake until firm, shriveled, and dry to the touch, about another 1 hour and 15 minutes. (During the last 30 minutes of cook time, check on chips often, and remove those that are done.)

0 point deviled egg

Ingredients [For 4 to 5 people]   [Preparation time : 12 minute – Cooking time : 15 minutes]

6 hard-boiled eggs

? cup of non-fat Greek yogurt

¼ tsp of Sriracha Sauce

2 scallions chopped

2 tablespoons of Fat-Free Cheddar Cheese (Kraft)

Preparation Method

Cut hard boiled eggs in half lengthwise and take the yolks out with a spoon.

Add the yolks to a medium-small sized bowl with the greek yogurt, sriracha sauce, scallions. Season with salt and pepper to taste.

Scoop the egg yolk mixture into the eggs and evenly divide the mixture.

Garnish the eggs with the cheddar cheese and more scallions if desired.

0 point sweet and sour grapes

Ingredients:

One large bunch of seedless grapes

1 Package of lime Jell-O (sugar free)

Directions:

Pour the Jell-O into a large bowl

Wash the grapes and give them a shake, but leave them really wet!

Pull the grapes off the vine and drop them into the bowl of Jell-O

Roll the grapes around in the bowl until they are coated

Put into Ziploc bags and place in the freezer until completely frozen (about 2 to 3 hours)

Enjoy!

0 point grilled fruit sticks

Ingredients:

½ of a honeydew melon (or cantaloupe) peeled, seeds removed

1 large (or 2 medium) ripe mangoes

About 12 medium strawberries, green tops cut off

1 Tablespoon of fresh mint leaves (optional)

4 Spray of a zero calorie cooking spray

Directions:

Cut the mango and honeydew into 1.5 inch squares (about 12 to 14 pieces total)

Put the fruit in alternating layers on 4 long skewers (about 9 pieces of fruit per skewer) If you only have wood skewers, soak them in water for 20-30 minutes before use

Coat your grill or grill pay with the cooking spray then turn on the flame to about medium high

Grill the skewers for about 2 minutes per side or until the fruit starts to show grill marks

Serve with fresh mint if desired

0 point Banana Pumpkin Bread

Ingredients:

1 Box of spice flavored cake mix

1 Can of pumpkin puree (15 ounce can)

3 or 4 ripe bananas, mashed well

Directions:

Preheat oven to 350 degrees

In a large mixing bowl, mix together all ingredients until well blended

Spray a loaf pan with zero calorie non-stick spray

Pour cake mixture into loaf pan

Bake for approximately 55 minutes or until toothpick comes out clean when inserted into the middle of the cake.

Serves 12

Twice Baked Zero Point Cauliflower

Ingredients:

1 large head of cauliflower, broken into pieces

¼ cup of low fat sour cream

½ cup sharp cheddar cheese, shredded

A dash of olive oil

Salt, pepper, and garlic powder to taste

Directions:

Preheat oven to 400 degrees

Rinse cauliflower and rip or cut into smaller pieces

Place in a large sauce pan and put approximately ¾ cup of water

Cover with lid and steam over low flame for about 12 minutes

Mash cauliflower with a potato masher

Add in sour cream, cheese, and seasonings

Add just enough olive oil to a Pyrex dish to coat it

Add the cauliflower mixture to the Pyrex dish

Bake for about 45 minutes or until crispy on top

Zippy Zero Point Brownies

Ingredients:

1 container of plain, nonfat Greek yogurt (6 ounces)

¼ cup of almond milk

3 tablespoons of Hershey special dark cocoa powder

2 scoops of any type or flavor of protein powder (whey powder is OK)

¼ cup of granulated artificial sweetener

1 egg

1/3 cup of canned pumpkin puree (or unsweetened applesauce)

1 teaspoon of baking powder

A pinch of salt

Directions:

Preheat oven to 400 degrees

Spray an 8X8 container with non-calorie cooking spray

Pour all ingredients into a large bowl and mix well

Pour batter into pan

Bake for approximately 15 to 20 minutes

Bean and Egg Muffins

Ingredients:

1.5 cups of canned black beans, drained and rinsed

1 green or red bell pepper, seeds removed and diced

1/2 cup of diced red onion

8 large eggs

Salt and pepper to taste

1 Jalapeno, seeds removed and diced (optional)

Directions:

Preheat oven to 350 degrees

Spray a skillet with a non-calorie cooking spray

Add the peppers, onion, and jalapeno, cooking under medium heat until tender (about 8 minutes)

Whisk together the eggs, add salt and pepper

Add the onions, peppers, and black beans to the eggs

Spray a muffin tin with the cooking spray

Pour egg mixture into each tin about 2/3's of the way full

Bake for 25 minutes or until each muffin is puffy and cooked all the way through (you can use a toothpick or knife to check for doneness)

Serve hot or cold or add to a freezer bag when completely cool

Easy Cauliflower Poppers

Ingredients:

1 Medium sized head of cauliflower

½ teaspoon of cumin

½ teaspoon of chili powder (more or less, depending on your taste)

½ teaspoon of seasoned salt

½ teaspoon of black pepper

Directions:

Preheat oven to 400 degrees

Coat a baking sheet liberally with a zero calorie cooking spray (butter flavor is good, but not necessary)

Cut your cauliflower into bite sized pieces (you should have about 4 cups, more or less)

Put the cauliflower in a medium bowl and add your spices

Mix until cauliflower is coated well

Put the cauliflower on the baking sheet, leaving room in-between pieces

Bake until cauliflower is soft, but not mushy (about 10 minutes or so)

An Almost Root Beer Float

Ingredients:

Fat free Whipped Topping (such as Cool Whip)

Diet Root Beer

Directions:

Put two big scoops (use your ice cream scoop!) of the frozen whipped topping in a tall glass or a bowl

Add ½ to 1 cup (or more) of root beer to the container

Chapter 8 : 1 Point recipes

Pancakes

Ingredients:

2 over-ripe bananas mashed

2 egg whites

1 cup of fat-free plain greek yogurt

1/2 cup of fat-free milk

1 teaspoon of pure vanilla extract

1 cup of all-purpose flour

2 teaspoons of baking powder

1/2 teaspoon of cinnamon

Instructions:

Preheat a nonstick electric skillet to 325 degrees.

In a medium sized bowl, combine mashed bananas, egg whites, greek yogurt, milk and vanilla extract. Whisk until well combines.

In a larger bowl, combine flour, baking powder and cinnamon and whisk.

Stir wet ingredient into dry ingredients.

Pour 1/4 cup of batter onto hot skillet and cook until golden brown.

Recipe Notes

To make blueberry pancakes, drop fresh blueberries into pancake batter once they are on the griddle

Banana Pancake Bites

Ingredients:

1 cup Bisquick Heart Smart Pancake & Baking Mix

2/3 cup skim milk

½ cup reduced calorie breakfast syrup

1 large ripe banana, chopped into small pieces

Directions:

Pre-heat the oven to 350. Lightly mist a 24 count mini muffin tin with cooking spray.

In a large bowl, stir together Bisquick mix, milk and syrup until thoroughly combined.

Divide the batter evenly amongst the prepared mini muffin tin cups. Sprinkle the chopped banana pieces over the tops of each muffin cup. Bake in the oven for 12-14 minutes until golden and cooked through.

Cloud Bread

Ingredients:

3 large eggs divided

1/8 tsp cream of tartar

3 tablespoons cream cheese or 1/3 cup fat free or light Greek yogurt

Instructions:

Preheat oven to 300 degrees F. Line a pan with parchment paper or a silpat mat.

Mix egg whites & cream of tartar on high speed until stiff peaks form.

In a large bowl mix egg yolks & greek yogurt (or cream cheese) until well combined and smooth. Gently fold in about 1 cup of the egg white mixture until well combined. Add remaining egg whites and fold just until mixed.

Divide egg mixture into 6 equal portions on prepared pan. Spread until about 1/2? thick.

Bake 30 minutes or until lightly browned. Immediately move to a wire rack and cool completely (at least 60 minutes).

Refrigerate in a sealed container to store.

Thai Chicken Skewers with Peanut Sauce

Ingredients:

Chicken & Marinade Ingredients:

3 tablespoons low sodium soy sauce

2 tablespoons honey

1 tablespoon sesame oil (found by the Asian sauces)

Juice from one lime

2 garlic cloves, minced

1 teaspoon Sriracha (Asian chili sauce found with the other Asian ingredients)

1/8 teaspoon of red pepper flakes

2 tablespoons chopped cilantro

1 ½ pounds (24 oz) raw boneless, skinless chicken breasts, cut into bite sized chunks

You'll also need 9" skewers – if using wooden skewers you should soak them in water for about 30 minutes before use

Peanut Sauce Ingredients:

2 tablespoons PB2 powdered peanut butter

1 tablespoon low sodium soy sauce

1 tablespoon water

1/8 teaspoon garlic powder

¼ teaspoon black pepper

1/8 teaspoon Sriracha

1 teaspoon brown sugar

1/8 teaspoon sesame oil

Directions:

To create the marinade, combine the soy sauce, honey, sesame oil, lime juice, garlic, sriracha, red pepper flakes and cilantro from the first set of ingredients and mix thoroughly. Pour marinade into a gallon Ziploc bag and add chicken. Seal bag and shake to coat chicken in the marinade. Place the bag in the refrigerator so that the chicken is covered in the marinade and refrigerate for at least 3-4 hours (but can marinate longer – i.e. all day, overnight, etc).

Pre-heat the grill until hot. Divide the chicken evenly onto the four skewers. Place the skewers on the grill over low heat. Depending on your grill, cooking times may vary. On our 4-burner grill the chicken skewers cooked in about 10 minutes, so I suggest cooking yours for about 5-6 minutes and then flipping them and continuing to cook until chicken is cooked through.

To make the sauce, place all sauce ingredients in a bowl and whisk together until combined. Serve each chicken skewer with about a tablespoon of peanut sauce for dipping.

easy cheesy garlic bread sticks

Ingredients:

1 cup of greek yogurt

1 cup of self rising flour

1 cup of part skim mozzarella cheese

1 tsp of basil

1 tsp of garlic powder

15 sprays of butter spray

Instructions:

In a medium bowl mix the greek yogurt and self rising flour until well combined.

Spread the dough out onto a floured works surface.

Coat a rolling pin with flour and begin to roll the dough out into an oval shape.

Transfer the dough onto a baking sheet and spritz the dough with butter spray.

In a small bowl combine the cheese, basil, and garlic powder. Spread the cheese on top of the dough and bake at 400 degrees for 15 minutes.

Serve with marinara sauce.

Super Healthy, Garlic Sauteed Spinach

Ingredients:

2 teaspoons olive oil

1 tablespoon garlic, minced (about 3 cloves)

1 (12 oz) bag baby spinach leaves

¼ teaspoon salt, or to taste

Fresh ground pepper, to taste

Fresh lemon

Instructions:

1. In a large, deep, nonstick pan or pot, heat olive oil. Add garlic and saute for 1 minute.

2. Add all spinach, salt, pepper and toss with garlic and oil. Cover pan and cook on low for about 1 minute. Uncover pan, turn the heat on high and cook spinach for another minute, or two, stirring with a wooden spoon until all the spinach is wilted.

3. Using a slotted spoon, lift the spinach into a serving dish or bowl and squeeze with a little fresh lemon all over the spinach.

4. Serve hot.

Makes 4 servings

Zucchini chips

Ingredients:

2 large zucchini

olive oil or PAM

Sea Salt

Instructions

Slice your Zucchini thinly

Arrange on a cookie sheet covered with foil or a baking stone

Place the Zucchini on the cookie sheet

Spray lightly with PAM or olive oil

Sprinkle lightly with Sea Salt

Bake at 250 degrees for 1 hour

Flip and Bake at 250 degrees for another hour

Make sure your chips are dried and turned into Zucchini Chips

Allow to cool and enjoy!

POINTS PLUS: 1 Point Per Serving

Chapter 9 : 2 Points recipes

Pizza Rolls

Ingredients:

8 egg roll wrappers (larger than wonton wrappers)

8 teaspoons store-bought pizza sauce

1 teaspoon Italian seasoning

24 turkey pepperoni slice

4 light Mozzarella string cheese sticks, each cut in half horizontally to make two shorter sticks

Directions:

Preheat the oven to 425. Lightly mist a large baking sheet with cooking spray and set aside.

Pour some water into a small dish and set aside. On a flat surface, place an egg roll wrapper, corner facing toward you (like a diamond) and spread a teaspoon of pizza sauce horizontally across the center of the wrapper, leaving ½ inch or so of space on each side. Sprinkle a pinch of Italian seasoning across the sauce and add a row of 3 pepperoni slices over the sauce. Place half a cheese stick on top of the pepperoni. Fold the bottom corner closest to you up over the ingredients and give it a 90 degree roll. Fold the side corners in and tuck them as you give the filled section another

90 degree roll. Dip your finger in the dish or reserved water and lightly wet the edges of the remaining top corner of the wrapper. Finish rolling the filled pizza log over the wet corner so that it adheres. Place wrapped pizza log onto the prepared baking sheet. Repeat with remaining ingredients.

When all of the pizza logs are wrapped and on the baking sheets, mist the tops with cooking spray. Bake for 10-14 minutes, flipping once halfway through, until the wrappers are golden brown.

Skinny Buffalo Ranch Tuna Salad

Prep Time: 10 minutes

Ingredients:

½ cup The Best Skinny Ranch Dressing or your favorite light ranch dressing

1 tablespoon hot buffalo wing sauce (I like Frank's Red Hot sauce), see shopping tips

A little cracked black pepper

2 (5 ounce) cans white meat tuna, packed in water and drained

¾ cup celery stalks, diced small

? cup carrots, diced small

Instructions:

1. Prepare The Best Skinny Ranch Dressing or use your favorite store bought light ranch dressing.

2. In a medium bowl, add drained tuna. Mash with a fork until flaky. To the tuna, add ranch dressing, hot buffalo wings sauce, black pepper, celery and carrots. Mix well until completely combined.

3. Store leftovers in a covered container in the fridge for up to 3 days.

Makes 2½ cups total.

Shopping Tips

I like to use sandwich thins when making sandwiches. Many brands can be found in most supermarkets. One sandwich thin has 100 calories, 1g fat, and 5g fiber.

I like Franks Red Hot Original sauce for this recipe. Many hot wings sauces are way too spicy for my taste. This one is just spicy enough. You'll find it in most supermarkets where Tabasco and other hot sauces are sold. Or, use your favorite sauce.

Serving Tips

To Make Sandwiches: Open each sandwich thin and spread ½ cup of tuna on the bottom of each. Top with 1 large slice of tomato. Top each with remaining half of sandwich thin. Makes 5 sandwiches, each ½ cup tuna salad

To Make Lettuce Wraps: Top each lettuce leaf with ¼ cup tuna salad and spread a little over the leaf. Top each lettuce wrap with a slice of tomato. Makes 10 lettuce wraps, each ¼ cup tuna salad (If serving for a meal, 2 lettuce wraps per person)

You can also serve as a dip with crackers.

taco soup

Ingredients:

1b lean ground beef 93/7 or lean ground turkey

1 medium Onion, diced

1 1oz packet Low Sodium Ranch Dressing Mix such as Mrs. Dash *see notes

1 1oz packet Low Sodium Taco Seasoning such as Mrs. Dash *see notes

1 32 oz. box (low sodium) Swanson Chicken Broth

14.5 oz. can Tomato Sauce (low sodium)

2 – 14.5 oz cans Diced Tomatoes with Chiles

14.5 oz can Black Beans, drained (low sodium)

1 can Corn, drained (low sodium)

Instructions:

Saute onions for 2 minutes.

Add ground beef and brown the meat.

Drain browned ground beef to remove excess fat.

Add ground beef mixture and all other ingredients to slow cooker.

Cook on High for 4 hours or Low for 6 hours.

Garnish with sour cream and cheddar cheese.

NOTES

SmartPoints: 2 (1 cup) (using lean ground turkey)

Smart Points: 3 93/7 ground beef

Makes about 10 servings

Turkey Sloppy Joes

Ingredients:

1 pound (454 grams) ground turkey breast (raw)

1 cup onion, diced

1/2 cup green pepper, diced

3 cloves garlic, minced

1 tablespoon yellow mustard

1/4 cup natural ketchup

1 (8 ounce) can no-salt added tomato sauce

1 tablespoon BBQ sauce

1-2 packets Stevia (optional, if you want to make it on the sweeter side)

Instructions:

Mist a skillet with oil and brown raw turkey, onions and green pepper over medium heat. (You could skip this step, but you will get a better flavor.)

Place turkey meat, onions & green pepper in the slow cooker. Add all the other ingredients and mix well.

Cover and cook on LOW for 3-4 hours or HIGH for 2-3 hours. If you don't brown the meat first, then cook on LOW for 5-6 hours or HIGH for 3-4 hours.

Serve with a whole grain bun, toasted.

Caramel cinnamon rolls – sugar free

Ingredients:

1 cup of self rising flour

1 cup of non fat greek yogurt

2 tablespoons of Erythritol (sugar substitute)

1 tsp of cinnamon

2 tablespoons of Sugar Free caramel sauce

15 sprays of butter spray

Instructions:

Preheat Oven to 350 degrees.

Combine flour and greek yogurt inside a mixing bowl and blend until ingredients have formed.

*if your dough still feels a little sticky, sprinkle flour onto dough until it feels solid and easy to separate.

Next, coat the cutting board with flour and lay the dough out on the cutting board. Using a rolling pin, roll the dough out to form a rectangular shape.

Spritz the dough 15 times with butter spray.

Sprinkle the dough with cinnamon and sugar

Roll the dough up so you have a long tube.

Cut the dough evenly into 8 equal pieces. Place the cinnamon rolls into an 8 inch cake pan and bake in the oven at 350 for 20 to 25 minutes. Take them out of the pan and pour 2 tablespoons of the sugar free caramel sauce over the cinnamon rolls. Enjoy!

Warm cinnamon swirls

Ingredients:

8 ounces reduced-fat crescent rolls

4 teaspoons sugar-cinnamon

1/2 cup powdered sugar

2 teaspoons skim milk

Instructions:

Unroll crescent dough; separate into 2 pieces. Press perforations together and sprinkle each with half of the sugar-cinnamon.Roll up 1 section, starting on long side and press firmly to eliminate air pockets. Pinch seam to seal. Cut each roll into 10 slices (For a total of 20 slices)Place rolls on baking sheet coated with cooking spray. Bake 10-12 minutes at 375 degrees.Once golden brown remove from oven. Whisk together powdered sugar and milk. Pour over warm rolls. Each roll is 1 weight watcher plus point. ONLY 1. I have to admit...I may or may not have eaten three while typing this point. These are great! Give them a try and let me know what you think! I have a feeling you won't be disappointed!

pizza bombs

Ingredients:

1 cup(s) fat-free plain Greek yogurt

1 cup(s) white self-rising flour

12 slice(s) turkey pepperoni

3 sticks of cheese

1oz parmesan cheese

2 tablespoons of light butter

1 tsp of garlic powder

Parsley flakes for garnish

Instructions:

Mix the greek yogurt and self rising flour in a medium size bowl until the dough starts to form. Cut the dough into 12 equal pieces.

Take one piece of dough and press each half into a circle with your thumb.

Place a pepperoni, and 1 cube of mozzarella on each dough.

Bring the edges up and over, pressing them together and being sure to leave no gaps for the filling to leak out. Lay the pizza bombs on a baking sheet lined with greased parchment paper

Combine melted butter, garlic, salt, and pepper in a small bowl. Brush the bombs with butter mixture onto each pizza bomb and top with parmesan.

Bake at 375 for 15-20 minutes.

Once pizza bombs are cool enough to handle, serve immediately. Enjoy!

Tortilla chips

Ingredients:

6 Mission Yellow Corn Tortillas Extra Thin

Non Stick Cooking Spray or Coconut Oil Spray

Kosher Salt

Instructions:

Preheat oven to 400 degrees.

Spray a baking sheet with non stick cooking spray.

Lay tortillas on baking sheet and spray both sides with cooking spray.

Stack tortillas and cut into 6 triangles.

Spread tortilla triangles into a single layer and bake, 6-9 minutes or until golden brown.

If baking two sheets of tortillas chips, rotate sheets halfway through baking.

Sprinkle with kosher salt and serve.

Recipe Notes

Tortillas chips will go from golden to overly browned very quickly. Check every minute for doneness after 6 minutes. Baking time can vary based on oven, if tortillas were chilled, even a darker baking pan may speed baking. Watch closely so they don't burn.

Chapter 10 : 3 Points recipes

Bagels

Ingredients:

To make 1 cup self rising flour sift together the follow:

1 cup flour

1 1/2 teaspoons baking powder

1/2 teaspoon salt

To make bagels:

1 cup of self rising flour

1 cup Fage Total 0% Greek Yogurt

1 Egg for egg wash

Instructions:

Preheat oven to 350 degrees.

Combine 1 cup of self rising flour and 1 cup of Fage Total 0% Greek Yogurt in a bowl until a dough starts to form.

Turn dough on a lightly floured surface and brush your hands with a bit of flour.

Knead and divide into 4 parts.

Roll out each dough ball to form a rope and pinch the ends of each rope together to make a circle. You will have four bagels.

Beat one egg and brush over the bagels .

Bake at 350 degrees on a pan sprayed with cooking spray for 23 minutes and 500 degrees for 2 minutes so the tops can brown

Cinnamon Applesauce pancakes recipe

Ingredients:

2 cups flour

4 teaspoons baking powder

2 cups water

2 tablespoons sugar

1/2 teaspoon salt

1/2 cup cinnamon applesauce

1/4 teaspoon vanilla extract

Preparation:

1. Combine dry ingredients, then add remaining ingredients and beat together.

2. Pour the batter onto a hot, lightly oiled griddle or skillet.

3. Cook until pancakes have a bubbly surface and slightly dry edges (2-3 minutes).

4. Turn pancakes. Cook for an additional 2-3 minutes (until golden brown).

Breakfast Burrito Bowl with Spiced Butternut Squash

Ingredients:

cooking spray

20-ounces butternut squash, seeded and cut into 1-inch cubes

1 1/2 teaspoons olive oil

3 teaspoons garlic powder

1/2 teaspoon cumin

1/2 teaspoon smoked paprika

3/4 teaspoon kosher salt

Freshly ground pepper, to taste

1 cup chopped tomatoes

1/3 cup chopped onion

1/4 cup chopped cilantro

Juice from ½ a lime

Olive oil spray

4 large eggs

4 ounces Hass avocado, cubed

1/4 cup reduced-fat shredded cheddar cheese

Directions:

Preheat oven to 425 degrees F. Spray a large nonstick baking sheet with oil. In a medium bowl, combine squash, olive oil, garlic powder, cumin, smoked paprika, 1/2 teaspoon salt and pepper. Toss well to coat. Spread squash evenly onto a sheet pan and roast for 20-25 minutes, or until browned and tender, tossing once halfway through.

Meanwhile, in a small bowl, combine tomatoes, onions, cilantro, lime juice, pinch of salt and pepper, to taste. Set aside.

Heat a small skillet over medium heat, lightly spray with olive oil spray, add eggs, season with salt, cover and cook to your desired doneness.

To assemble bowls: Layer 2/3 cup squash, 1/2 cup pico, 1 oz avocado, 1 egg and 1 tablespoon cheese. Repeat for remaining bowls.

Crockpot Stuffed Pepper Soup Recipe

Ingredients:

1 lb extra lean ground turkey or beef

1 cup onion , chopped

14.5 oz can diced tomatoes with roasted garlic and onions

15 oz can tomato sauce

2 cups green and red peppers , chopped (I've added up to four peppers, and it's yummy!)

3 cups beef broth

½ teaspoon basil

1.5 packets of chili seasoning

1 cup cooked rice , brown or white

Instructions:

Brown ground beef with onion in a skillet over medium heat.

Drain beef and onions and place in crock pot.

Chop peppers, add to crock pot.

Add tomatoes (including juice) and remaining ingredients, except rice – which should be added 1 hour before end of cooking.

Cover and cook on low for 6-8 hours.

Egg Drop Soup with Chicken

Ingredients:

4 cup low sodium chicken broth, (use a good quality stock)

1/2 tsp soy sauce

1/2 cup cooked boneless, skinless chicken breast, chopped

1/2 cup frozen green peas, (baby peas are nice)

1/4 cup green onion, thinly sliced

1 egg, lightly beaten

Directions:

Prep 5 min Cook 5 min Ready 10 min

In saucepan, bring chicken stock and soy sauce to a boil. Add chicken, peas and green onion; bring to a boil again.

Remove from heat; drizzle in egg in slow steady stream. Let sit for 1 minute for egg to set.

Stir gently before ladling into bowls.

Per serving: 3 SmartPoints; 3 PointsPlus; 2 POINTS (old)

Recipe originally inspired by Food.com with 5-star rating and 12 reviews.

Chicken salad with Apples and Cranberries

Ingredients:

2 1/2 cups chopped cooked chicken

3 stalks celery, chopped

1 cup chopped apple, about 1 large; I used a Pink Lady and kept the peel because it was organic

1/4 cup dried cranberries

1/2 cup nonfat plain Greek yogurt

2 tablespoons of light mayonnaise

2 teaspoons lemon juice

2 tablespoons chopped parsley (optional)

Salt and pepper to taste

Instructions:

Place the chicken, celery, apple and cranberries in a bowl and stir to combine and then set it aside.

In a small bowl, stir together the yogurt, mayonnaise and lemon juice.

Add this to the chicken mixture and stir to mix well.

Stir in the parsley if desired. Season to taste with salt and pepper.

Veggie ranch pizza

Ingredients:

2 8 ounces (226g) reduced-fat cream cheese, softened

1 (1 ounce/28g) package powdered Ranch dressing mix

2 (8 ounces/226g) cans reduced-fat Pillsbury Crescent Rolls

1 cup (91g) fresh broccoli, chopped

1 cup (175g) fresh red pepper, chopped

4 green onions, chopped

1 1/2 cups (120g) shredded cheddar cheese

Instructions:

Preheat oven to 350°F.

Place cream cheese, and Ranch dressing mix in a large bowl. With an electric mixer, beat on medium until smooth and creamy. Set aside. You can soften cream cheese in microwave so that it's easier to mix with the ranch.

Remove crescent rolls from the cans and roll out in one big piece onto a large, greased cookie sheet. Pinch seams together, if needed. Bake for 8-10 minutes or until golden brown. Let cool.

Spread cream cheese mixture onto cooled crust. Top with cheese and veggies.

Use a pizza cutter or large knife to cut into squares. Serve immediately or store in refrigerator in airtight container for up to 3 or 4 days.

Parmesan Chicken Cutlets

Ingredients:

1/4 cup parmesan cheese, grated

2 tbsp dried seasoned Italian bread crumbs

1/8 tsp paprika

1 tsp dried parsley

1/2 tsp garlic powder

1/4 tsp black pepper, freshly ground

4 boneless chicken breast, about 1 pound

Directions:

Prep 10 min Cook 25 min Ready 35 min

Preheat oven to 400 degrees.

In resealable plastic bag, combine cheese, crumbs and all seasonings; shake well.

Transfer mixture to plate; dip each chicken breast in cheese mixture, turning to coat all sides.

Arrange on nonstick baking sheet.

Bake until chicken is cooked through, 20-25 minutes.

Per serving: 3 SmartPoints; 4 PointsPlus; 4 POINTS (old)

Lemon Pepper Chicken Breasts

Ingredients:

2 tbsp lemon pepper seasoning,

1 tbsp all-purpose flour

4 (3 oz each) boneless, skinless chicken breast

1 tbsp unsalted butter

1/2 medium lemon, zested and juiced

1 cup low-sodium chicken broth

Directions:

Prep 10 min Cook 25 min Ready 35 min

On a large plate, combine lemon pepper seasoning with flour. Pat chicken dry and coat with flour mixture. Heat butter in a large skillet, add chicken, and brown for about 3 minutes per side.

Mix together lemon zest and juice with broth. Pour over chicken, cover, and cook for 15 minutes. Remove lid and cook for another 5 minutes or until juices run clear.

Per serving: 3 SmartPoints; 3 PointsPlus; 3 POINTS (old)

Skillet Lemon Chicken with Olives and Herbs

Ingredients:

1/2 tbsp extra virgin olive oil

4 (8 oz) boneless chicken breasts

1/2 tsp kosher salt

2 teaspoons all purpose or gluten free flour

2 cloves garlic, crushed

1/2 cup dry white wine

1/4 cup lemon juice

1 teaspoon lemon zest

1 teaspoon chopped fresh thyme

1 cup pitted chopped olives

1 tbsp chopped fresh parsley

optional, 4 thin lemon slices

Directions:

Preheat oven to 400F with the rack in the center position.

Heat the oil in a 10 inch cast iron skillet over medium-high heat. Season chicken with salt and pepper then sprinkle with flour. When oil is hot, sear chicken about 3 minutes on each side.

Add garlic, wine, lemon zest, lemon juice, thyme and olives. Top with lemon slices if desired, transfer the pan to the oven and bake about 10 minutes, until 165F in the center.

Serve hot topped with parsley

Oven Fried Pork Chops

Ingredients:

6 oz center-cut lean pork loin chop

2 tbsp pineapple juice

1 tbsp low-sodium soy sauce

1/4 tsp ground ginger

1/8 tsp garlic powder

1 large egg white, lightly beaten

1/3 cup dry bread crumbs

1/4 tsp dried Italian seasoning

1/4 tsp paprika

1 dash garlic powder

1 cooking spray

Directions:

Prep 15 min Cook 50 min Ready 65 min

Preheat oven to 350 degrees.

Trim fat from chops.

Combine juice, soy sauce, ginger, garlic powder and egg whites in a bowl; stir well.

Combine breadcrumbs, Italian seasoning, paprika, and dash of garlic powder in a shallow dish; stir well.

Dip chops in juice mixture, and dredge in breadcrumbs mixture.

Place chops on a broiler pan coated with cooking spray.

Bake at 350 degrees for 50 minutes or until tender, turning after 25 minutes.

Per serving: 3 SmartPoints; 3 PointsPlus; 3 POINTS (old)

Oven Baked Onion Rings

Ingredients:

Canola oil spray

4 cups baked potato chips

1/2 tsp. cayenne pepper

1 cup low-fat buttermilk

1/2 cup plus 2 Tbs. all-purpose flour

1/2 tsp. salt, plus more to taste

1/4 tsp. freshly ground black pepper

1 to 2 large Vidalia onions, peeled

Chapter 11 : 4 points recipes

4 point Baked Vegetable Omelet

Ingredients:

1/2 cup red onion, diced small

1/2 cup green bell pepper, diced small

1 cup baby spinach, roughly chopped

5 egg whites

2 eggs

1/4 cup skim milk

1/2 teaspoon Kosher salt

1/4 teaspoon ground black pepper

1/2 cup low-fat cheddar cheese, shredded

Instructions:

Preheat oven to 375 degrees. Spray a 9 x 13 inch casserole pan with nonstick spray.

Combine all ingredients and mix well until eggs are frothy and vegetables are well distributed. Pour into prepared pan and sprinkle the cheese on top. Bake for about 40 minutes until egg is set and lightly browned. If the top is beginning to brown too quickly, remove and cover with foil. Continue baking until set.

Allow to rest for 10 minutes before slicing and serving, enjoy!

Pineapple French Toast 4 point

Ingredients:

1medium egg

1/4tsp.cinnamon, divided

1/4cup canned crushed pineapple, no sugar added

1 slice raisin bread

Directions:

In a shallow dish, beat the egg and 1/8 tsp. cinnamon. Drain juice from pineapple into egg mixture; beat again. Prick both sides of bread with a fork. Soak bread in egg mixture, turning several times until as much egg mixture as possible is absorbed. Carefully transfer to a nonstick baking sheet. Combine drained pineapple and remaining 1/8 tsp. cinnamon with any leftover egg mixture. Spread on top of bread. Bake at 400Â° for 20 minutes. Makes 1 serving

Bake for 60 minutes, or until the center is set.

Crustless Spinach Quiche with Sun-Dried Tomatoes 4 point

Ingredients:

Quiche

6 eggs

6 egg whites

2 cups loosely packed spinach, coarsely chopped

1/4 cup freshly grated parmesan cheese

1/2 cup chopped sun-dried tomatoes with no liquid (reconstituted according to package directions, if necessary)

1/2 cup chopped onion

1 clove garlic, minced

1 tablespoon olive oil

1/4 teaspoon kosher or sea salt

1/4 teaspoon black pepper

Crust (optional)

3/4 cups whole wheat pastry flour

1/4 cup oat flour using 1/4 cup rolled oats* see directions

1/4 teaspoon kosher or sea salt

1/3 cup coconut oil, cold and solid but scoopable, refrigerate prior (optional, pure unsalted butter)

2- 3 tablespoons ice cold water

2 tablespoons walnut pieces, optional

Instructions:

Preheat oven to 375 degrees.

For the crust:

Place rolled oats in a food processor or blender and pulse until a coarse flour is created.

Mix together the oat flour with the whole wheat flour and salt. Add the coconut oil in in small pieces at a time.

Blend with a pastry cutter or hands or pulse in the food processor until pea like crumbles are in the crust. Add the water in small amounts until dough is the right consistency: Dough should be pretty shaggy and dry but come together when pinched between the forefinger and thumb.

Form the dough into a ball. Wrap tightly in plastic wrap and refrigerate for 30 minutes and up to 24 hours. Don't worry if dough is shaggy, it will come together more after refrigeration. Roll dough out onto a floured work surface. Place the quiche/pie pan on top of the dough, upside down, and cut a circle. Carefully turn over and press the dough into the pie pan and trim the edges.

Use a fork to crimp the outer edges of the crust or use fingers and fold over edges. Add the quiche mixture (recipe below).

For the quiche filling:

Heat onion and garlic in a skillet with olive oil for about 5 minutes, until onion is softened and translucent. Add spinach and cook, just until wilted. Remove from heat. Mix in sun-dried tomatoes.

Meanwhile, beat/whisk egg whites until very frothy. Whisk whole eggs in a separate bowl. Combine the eggs and whites. Add parmesan cheese, salt, and pepper. Fold in the spinach tomato mixture and pour into the pie shell. Bake for 25 minutes or until set in the center and golden at the edges.

If desired, sprinkle with walnut pieces 5 minutes before removing from the oven.

Blueberry oatmeal muffins recipe

Ingredients:

1 1/2 cups quick-cooking oats

2/3 cup all-purpose flour

1/2 cup whole-wheat flour

1/2 cup packed light brown sugar

1 tsp ground cinnamon

1 tsp ground nutmeg

1 tsp baking powder

1 tsp baking soda

3/4 teaspoon salt

1 cup fat free buttermilk

1/4 cup canola oil

1 tsp vanilla

2 tsp lemon zest

1/2 cup liquid egg substitute (like EggBeaters)

2 cups fresh blueberries

Instructions:

Preheat oven to 400°.

Place oats in a food processor; pulse 5 to 6 times or until oats resemble coarse meal. Place in a large bowl.

Add in flours, baking soda, baking powder, salt, sugar, cinnamon and nutmeg; stir well.

In a separate bowl, combine buttermilk, oil, vanilla, lemon zest and liquid egg substitute. Then add to flour mixture; stir just until moist.

Gently fold blueberries into batter. Spoon batter into 16 muffin cups coated with cooking spray.

Bake at 400° for 20 minutes or until muffins spring back when touched lightly in center.

Remove from pans immediately; place on a wire rack.

Preparation time: 10 minute(s)

Cooking time: 20 minute(s)

Diet type: Vegetarian

avocado toast with sunny side egg 4 point

Ingredients:

1 slice whole grain bread, toasted (1.5 oz)

1 oz mashed (1/4 small haas) avocado

cooking spray

1 large egg

kosher salt and black pepper to taste

hot sauce (optional)

Directions:

Mash the avocado in a small bowl and season with salt and pepper.

Heat a small nonstick skillet over low heat, spray with oil and gently crack the egg into the skillet. Cover and cook to your liking.

Place mashed avocado over toast, top with egg, salt and pepper and hot sauce if desired!

Chapter 12 : 5 Points recipes

lunch power muesli

Ingredients:

1 cup rye flakes

1 cup wheat germ

3/4 cup oat rolled date pieces, coarsely chopped

3/4 cup raisins

1/2 cup chia seeds

1/2 cup sliced almonds

2 tablespoons coconut palm sugar

1 teaspoon ground cinnamon

1/2 teaspoon sea salt

Instructions:

If oat-rolled date pieces are large, coarsely chop. Otherwise, combine all ingredients in a large glass bowl and mix until well combined.

Store in an airtight container for 3 weeks to a month. Alternately, store in freezer for up to 3 months.

breakfast sandwich 5 point

Ingredients:

1 100 Calorie Sandwich Thins

1 large egg

1/2 tsp salt

1/4 tsp pepper

1 slice fat-free American cheese

1/4 cup chopped spinach leaves

1 slice lean deli ham

2 slices fresh tomato

1 slice red onion

Instructions:

Spray a small frying pan with non-stick cooking spray and set to medium heat.

Toast your Sandwich Round in a toaster.

While bread is toasting, fry the slice of ham until it edges start to become a bit crisp. Place ham on 1 half of the toasted Sandwich Round.

Next, add the spinach to the frying pan, and cover with a lid until the leaves start to wilt (about 1 minute).

Add in egg, salt and pepper. Scramble egg whites with spinach and cook until egg is solid.

Pile up the eggs into one section of the pan, and top with the slice of cheese. Cover pan with lid, and turn off heat. After about 30 seconds, remove the lid and cheese should be melted.

Place eggs with the cheese on top of the ham on your sandwich.

Finally, top with tomatoes, onions and the remaining half of the Sandwich Round.

Lemon Poppy Seed Pancakes

Ingredients:

6 oz container of lemon flavored non-fat Greek yogurt (I used Chobani)

1 large egg

1 tablespoon honey

zest from one large lemon

½ cup of white whole wheat flour (you can use all-purpose or wheat, this is just my preference)

1 teaspoon baking soda

1 teaspoon poppy seeds

Optional (for strawberry topping):

8 medium strawberries, sliced

½ teaspoon fresh lemon juice

1 tablespoon powdered sugar

Directions:

In a large mixing bowl, combine the yogurt, egg, honey and lemon zest and stir until thoroughly combined. Add the flour, baking soda and poppy seeds and stir until batter is mixed.

In a small bowl, combine sliced strawberries, lemon juice and powdered sugar and mix until sugar is dissolved. Set aside.

Lightly mist a griddle pan with cooking spray and bring over medium heat. Scoop ¼ cup of batter onto the heated pan and use the back of a spoon to smooth it out into a flat circle. Repeat in batches (depending on how many pancakes fir on your pan at once) to form 6 pancakes. Cook on one side for 2-4 minutes until bottom is golden and pancake is "flappable." If the batter is not firm on the bottom yet it needs more time. Once flipped cook another 1-2 minutes until golden on the other side as well. Repeat until you have 6 pancakes. Each serving is 2 pancakes with 1/3 of the strawberry topping.

Egg and Bacon Stuffed Acorn Squash 5 point

Ingredients:

1 large (about 4-inch) acorn squash

1 tablespoon olive oil

1/4 teaspoon kosher salt

1/4 teaspoon ground black pepper

4 large eggs

1/4 teaspoon dried thyme leaves

2 slices turkey bacon, cooked and crumbled

Instructions:

Preheat oven to 425. Line a large baking sheet with parchment paper and set aside.

Trim off the ends of the square and discard. Slice the squash width-wise into 4 equal round slices. Remove the seeds from the center of each.

Brush both sides of the squash rings with the olive oil and season with the salt and pepper. Place on the prepared baking sheet and bake for 15 minutes or until tender.

Remove from the oven and reduce the oven temperature to 350. Crack an egg into the center of each acorn slice and bake for 12 minutes or until eggs are cooked. Sprinkle with thyme and bacon. Serve and enjoy!

Chapter 13 : 6 Points recipes

Blueberry Cheese Danish

Ingredients:

2 Slices 35 Calorie Bread

4 TBS. Whipped Cream Cheese

1/2 cup fresh blueberries

1/4 tsp. Truvia 0 calorie sweetener

Directions:

Lightly toast bread slices. Spread 2 TBS. cream cheese on each slice. Evenly distribute blueberries on each slice. Sprinkle with Truvia. Place under broiler for 2-3 minutes (until blueberries are about to burst).

Potato Soup

Ingredients:

1   (26 to 30-ounce) bag frozen hash browns

2   (14-ounce) cans non-fat chicken broth

1   (10.75-ounce) can 98% fat-free cream of chicken soup

1/4   cup onion, chopped

1/4   teaspoon black pepper

1   (8-ounce) package low-fat cream cheese

1   cup fat-free milk

Green onions, chopped, to garnish

Bacon bits, optional, to garnish

Directions:

Add hash browns, chicken broth, chicken soup, onion, and black pepper to your slow-cooker and cook on high for an hour. Stir, then turn your slow-cooker to low for another hour.

Add cream cheese, and cook another 1/2 hour or until cheese can be stirred into the mixture.

Add milk and cook 10 to 15 minutes longer.

Garnish with chopped green onion and bacon bits. Add 1 WW point for garnish.

VARIATIONS:

Use frozen country potatoes or Potatoes O'Brien in place of the hash browns.

Creamy Chicken & Wild Rice Soup

Ingredients:

2 cups water

4 cups (32 oz) less sodium fat free chicken broth

1 lb raw boneless skinless chicken breasts

1 (6 oz) box of Long Grain & Wild Rice (I used Uncle Ben's) – not the quick cooking kind, do not prepare

1 cup sliced or diced carrots

1 cup sliced celery

½ cup flour

½ teaspoon salt

½ teaspoon black pepper

1 stick (8 tablespoons) light butter (I used Land O'Lakes)

2 cups fat free half and half

Directions:

Bring the water and chicken broth to a boil in a large pot or dutch oven. Add the chicken, rice (with seasoning packet), carrots and celery and reduce heat to a simmer. Cover the pot and simmer for 25-30 minutes until chicken is cooked through and easy to shred.

Remove the cooked chicken breasts to a plate and shred with two forks. Replace the lid and continue to simmer the rest.

Mix together the flour, salt and pepper in a bowl until combined. In a medium saucepan, melt the butter over medium heat. Stir in flour a spoonful at a time to make a roux. Pour the half and half in a little at a time, stirring continuously with a whisk to allow the roux to combine with the cream. Continue whisking and adding half and half until the mixture is smooth and creamy.

Add the shredded chicken and the cream mixture back into the soup pot and stir to combine. Bring back to a simmer and simmer for 5-10 minutes to allow soup to thicken and flavors to combine.

Skinny Chicken Nuggets

Ingredients:

3 chicken breasts fillets, skinless, cut into 1" cubes

2 cups Panko bread crumbs, (whole wheat can be found at any whole foods type supermarket and most organic sections of your local grocery)

1 large egg white, lightly whipped

1 tablespoon Extra-Virgin Olive Oil or Canola Oil

1 teaspoon black pepper

1/8 teaspoon cayenne pepper

1/4 teaspoon onion powder

Salt to taste

Instructions:

Preheat oven to 400 degrees. In a large bowl add egg white and chicken cubes, toss to coat. Add seasonings to chicken along with Panko bread crumbs, coat well. It may be necessary to press crumbs onto chicken pieces. Place chicken coated pieces on a non-stick cookies sheet, drizzle with oil or use an oil sprayer if available. Cook 30 minutes until chicken is cooked through.

Bacon ranch Turkey Wrap

Ingredients:

4 Flatout Light Original flatbreads

8 slices bacon

8 oz roasted turkey deli meat

4 slices fat free American cheese (I used Kraft brand)

1 tomato (thinly sliced)

Red onion slices

1/4 cup light ranch dip or dressing

Iceberg or Romaine lettuce

Instructions:

Spread ranch dressing all over the center of the flatbread.

Top with turkey, bacon, lettuce, cheese, onion, and tomatoes. Fold the sides in, and then roll up.

2 pizza bread

Ingredients:

To make 2 balls of dough:

1/2 cup self rising flour

1/2 cup Fage Total 0% fat free Greek Yogurt

For Pizza:

1/3 cup Kirkland Marinara sauce

2 oz Trader Joe's Lite Shredded Mozzarella cheese

Instructions:

Preheat oven to 450 degrees.

Combine self rising flour and Greek yogurt to make the dough.

Divide into two equal pieces. You can freeze one and use the other.

Turn the dough you will be using onto a floured surface and knead.

Roll out dough and place in a small greased pizza pan.

Bake for 5 minutes at 450. Keep an eye out for it not to get too brown.

Remove from oven and top with sauce and cheese.

Return to oven and bake for another 10 minutes, checking to make sure it doesn't get too dark.

Taco Casserole

Ingredients:

1 lb ground chicken breast or turkey

1/2 diced white onion

1 can whole kernel corn

1 can black beans

1 tbsp taco seasoning

2 tbsp taco sauce

1/4 cup fat free sour cream

1/2 cup fat free shredded cheddar cheese

1 cup diced fresh tomatoes

1/3 cup green onions

Directions:

Saute meat, beans, onions, taco seasoning, sauce, and corn on medium-high heat until meat is browned (or soy crumbles are thoroughly cooked).

Spoon half your meat mixture into your casserole dish in an even layer, top with a thin layer of sour cream, then sprinkle with some cheese.

Repeat. Cover with cheese.

Bake at 350 for 15 minutes, then serve topped with diced tomatoes and green onions.

Sheet pan lemon Rosemary chicken and potatoes

Ingredients:

3 Tbsp olive oil, divided

1 Tbsp lemon juice

Zest of 1 lemon

2 cloves garlic, minced

1 Tbsp fresh rosemary, chopped

1 Tbsp fresh thyme, chopped

1½ tsp. sea salt

1 tsp. black pepper

4 boneless, skinless chicken breasts

3 cups baby red potatoes, quartered

1 lb. fresh green beans

Instructions:

Preheat oven to 400 degrees F.

In a small bowl, whisk together 2 tablespoons olive oil, lemon juice, zest, garlic, rosemary, thyme, salt and pepper. In a separate bowl toss together potatoes with tablespoon olive oil and season with additional salt and pepper, if desired.

On a large baking sheet lightly sprayed with oil, arrange chicken breasts, potatoes and green beans and drizzle herb mixture over top, using a brush or your hands to make sure everything is evenly coated.

Place the pan in the oven and roast for 25 to 30 minutes, depending on the size of your breasts. Chicken should have an internal temp of 165 degrees F, potatoes should be tender and green beans nice and crisp! Feel free to turn the broiler on for a couple minutes if you like your potatoes a bit more crisp.

Serve and enjoy!

Sour Cream and Onion Chicken

Ingredients:

4 chicken breast halves

1 12 oz can of low fat cream of mushroom soup

1/2 cup fat free sour cream

1 1/2 cups water1 packet of onion soup mix

Directions:

Minutes to prepare: 30 | Minutes to cook 320

Notes: This has got to be one of the easiest meals to put together and has become a family favorite. It's very creamy and goes well with wild rice or potatoes. The recipe doubles nicely for larger servings.

Chicken Fried Steaks

Ingredients:

4 lean cube steaks

1/2 cup fat-free buttermilk

1 cup flour (reserve 1 Tablespoon)

1 teaspoon salt

1 teaspoon McCormick's Montreal steak seasoning

2 tablespoons oil

2 cups skim milk

Directions:

1. Dip steaks in buttermilk. Combine flour, salt, and steak seasoning (remember to keep 1

tablespoon set aside). Dip steaks in flour mixture.

2. Set steaks on wax paper, let set for 20 minutes.

3. Heat 1 tablespoons oil in skillet, add steaks, cook until both sides are golden brown.

Remove from pan and keep warm.

4. Combine milk and reserved TBSP of flour in bowl until well mixed.

5. Stirring constantly, add milk mixture to skillet. Once added, bring mixture to a boil.

6. Lower heat and simmer until gravy thickens.

7. Serve over steaks.

Skinny Chimichangas

Ingredients Serves 4

1/2 lb ground turkey breast

1 onion, finely chopped

1 clove garlic, minced

2 tsp chili powder

1 tsp dried oregano

1/2 tsp ground cumin

1 can (8 oz) tomato sauce

2 tbsp mild green chili pepper, chopped

1/3 cup reduced-fat cheddar cheese, shredded

4 (8 inch each) fat-free flour tortillas

Directions:

Prep 15 min Cook 40 min Ready 55 min

Preheat the oven to 400 degrees F.

Spray a nonstick baking sheet with nonstick spray; set aside.

Spray a medium nonstick skillet with nonstick spray; set over medium-high heat.

Add the turkey, onion, garlic, chili powder, oregano, and cumin.

Cook, breaking up the turkey with a wooden spoon until browned, about 6 miuntes.

Stir in the tomato sauce and the chiles; bring to a boil.

Reduce the heat and simmer, uncovered, until the flavors are blended and the mixture thickens, slightly, about 5 minutes.

Remove from the heat and stir in the cheddar cheese.

Meanwhile, wrap the tortillas in foil and place in the oven to warm for 10 minutes.

Spoon about 1/2 cup of the filling into the center of each tortilla.

Fold in the sides, then roll to enclose the filling.

Place the chimichangas, seam-side down, on the baking sheet.

Lightly spray the tops of the tortillas with nonstick spray.

Bake until golden and crisp, about 20 minutes. Do not turn.

Per serving: 6 SmartPoints; 5 PointsPlus; 4 POINTS (old)

Meatloaf

Ingredients:

2 teaspoons canola oil

1 cup finely chopped white mushrooms

1 cup finely chopped onion

1 carrot, peeled and finely chopped

1 stalk celery, finely chopped

1 pound lean ground beef (7% or less)

1/2 cup quick cooking or old-fashioned oats (not instant)

2 large egg whites (I use 1 whole egg instead)

3 tablespoons ketchup (plus more for brushing on top)

1 tablespoon Worcestershire sauce

1 teaspoon dried thyme leaves (not ground thyme)

1 teaspoon salt

1/4 teaspoon black pepper

1/2 teaspoon garlic powder (or 1 teaspoon minced fresh)

Instructions:

Preheat oven to 350F degrees. Spray a 4-1/2 x 8-1/2-inch loaf pan with cooking spray.

Heat the oil in a large nonstick skillet set over medium heat. Add the mushrooms, onion, carrot, and celery. Cook, stirring frequently, until the onion is softened, about 5 minutes. Transfer this mixture to a large bowl.

Add the remaining ingredients to the vegetables in the bowl and mix well. Press the meatloaf into the prepared loaf pan.

Bake the meatloaf for 30 minutes. Brush additional ketchup on top of the loaf, if desired.

Cook until done, an additional 30 to 45 minutes. (An instant read thermometer inserted into the center of the loaf should read 160F degrees.)

Remove from the oven and let rest for about 5 minutes. Cut into 8 slices.

Chapter 14 : 7 Points recipes

Lasagna soup

Ingredients:

1 yellow onion, chopped

kosher salt

1 lb. lean ground turkey sausage (I used Jennie-O) or 93% lean ground beef (points will be different!)

4 cloves garlic, minced

28 oz. can crushed tomatoes or 28 oz jar of marinara sauce

1 tbsp. dried oregano

5 c. low-sodium chicken broth

8 oz. lasagna noodles, broke into 2? pieces

2 c. low fat shredded mozzarella

Toppings (optional):

Grated Parmesan, for garnish

Torn fresh basil, for garnish

Instructions:

In a large skillet over medium heat, spray the bottom of the pan with cooking spray. Add onions and season with salt. Cook until tender and golden, 5 minutes, then add sausage and cook until no longer pink. Drain fat and return to pot.

Add garlic and stir until fragrant, 1 minute, then add crushed tomatoes and dried oregano.

Pour in chicken broth and bring to a simmer.

Add lasagna noodles and cook, stirring occasionally, until al dente, 10 minutes.

Add mozzarella and stir, letting melt into soup.

Garnish with Parm and basil.

Apple Cheddar Turkey Wraps

Ingredients:

1 Flatout Light Original Flatbread

1-2 leaves green leaf lettuce, torn

2 oz thinly sliced deli turkey

1 oz sliced 50% reduced fat sharp cheddar cheese

1 ½ teaspoons apple cider vinegar

½ teaspoon canola oil

½ teaspoon honey

A pinch of salt and pepper

¼ cup matchstick-sliced apple pieces (slice apple into thin, short sticks)

1/3 cup coleslaw mix (just the shredded veggies, undressed)

Directions:

Lay the Flatout flatbread on a clean, dry surface and lay the torn lettuce down the center of the flatbread going the long way (starting at the rounded end and spreading down the length of the flatbread to the other rounded end). You can leave a bit of space at each end as you'll be folding them over, and you do not need to cover the whole flatbread, just an area down the middle. Top the lettuce with the sliced deli turkey and the cheddar cheese.

In a small mixing bowl, combine the vinegar, oil, honey, salt and pepper and stir until well combined. Add the apples and coleslaw and stir to coat. Lay the apple/coleslaw mixture on top of the other ingredients layered on the wrap.

Fold in the rounded ends of the flatbread over the filling. Then fold one of the long edges over the filling and continue to roll until the wrap is completely rolled up. Cut in half and serve.

Scrumptuous Chicken Fried Rice

Ingredients:

1½ cups cooked chicken breast, skinless and diced

3½ cups cooked brown rice, you can use about 1 cup rawBasmati brown rice

1½ tbsp canola oil

1 cup frozen peas, unthawed

½ cup sliced scallions

2 tsp toasted sesame oil or canola oil

1 cup chopped celery

3 tbsp low-sodium soy sauce

4 egg whites

2 scallions for garnish (optional)

black pepper, to taste

Instructions:

1. Add canola oil in a large nonstick pan or nonstick wok and preheat over medium-high heat. Mix in cooked chicken and scallions and stir-fry for about 1 minute.

2. Add the broken frozen peas, cooked rice, celery, and soy sauce. Cook for around 3 minutes until heated through, stir softly to coat all ingredients. Move rice mixture to the sides of pan or wok. Add egg whites to the center of wok. Cook while stirring about

1 minute or until the egg whites are fully cooked. Mix together eggs and rice mixture. Pour sesame oil, a bit black pepper and then stir fry ingredients all together.

3. You can serve immediately. Leftovers can be stored in a refrigerator during the next 2 days.

Chicken pasta

Ingredients:

1/2 lb whole wheat penne pasta

4 slice bacon, diced

1/2 Tbsp light butter

1 large chicken breast, boneless & skinless, cut into bite sized pieces

1 Tbsp all purpose flour

1/2 pkg ranch dressing mix (1/2 oz)

1 c fat free milk

1/2 c fat free shredded cheddar cheese

salt & pepper to taste

Instructions:

Cook pasta according to package directions in boiling salted water; drain, return to pot, and keep warm.

Meanwhile, cook bacon in a large skillet over medium heat until crisp. Drain on paper towels. Drain all but 1/2 tablespoon of bacon drippings from the pan.

Season the chicken with salt and pepper. Add the butter to the reserved bacon drippings, then add the chicken to the same skillet. Cook until tender, no longer pink, and slightly browned.

Sprinkle the flour and ranch dressing mix over the chicken, stirring to coat evenly. Stir in the milk, and cook, stirring occasionally, until thickened and bubbly. Stir in the cheddar cheese and half of the reserved bacon; cook and stir until the cheese is melted. Taste for seasoning and adjust as needed.

Serve each plate of pasta with more bacon sprinkled over the top.

Stuffed Cabbage Rolls

Ingredients:

For the rolls:

12 leaves cabbage

1 cup cooked long grain rice

1 egg, beaten

1/4 cup milk

1/4 cup finely chopped white or yellow onion

1 clove finely chopped garlic

1 pound raw, lean ground turkey

For the sauce:

1 1/4 teaspoons salt

1 1/4 teaspoons ground black pepper

1 (15-ounce) can tomato sauce

2 tablespoons ketchup

1 teaspoon Worcestershire sauce

1 teaspoon paprika

2 tablespoons lemon juice

2 tablespoons honey

1/2 teaspoon dried thyme leaves

Instructions:

Bring a pot of salted water to a boil over high heat. Boil cabbage leaves for 2 minutes. Whisk together tomato sauce, honey, spices, lemon juice, ketchup, the salt and pepper, and Worcestershire sauce.

In a separate bowl, combine the cooked rice, egg, milk, onion, garlic, and ground turkey. Add in 1/4 of the sauce and combine well.

Scoop about 1/4 cup of the gound turkey mix into the center of each cabbage roll. Roll up the leaves, tucking in the ends. Top with tomato sauce and cover.

Cook on low for 8 to 9 hours or on high for 4 to 5 hours.

Taco Fiesta bubble up casserole

Ingredients:

1 lb cooked extra lean ground beef

1 7.5oz package pillsbury biscuits, (10 biscuits to the pack, the ones In the 4 value pack, if you can't find that size you can buy the bigger size and weigh it out)

Taco seasoning (I buy a store bought 30g pack)

1? cup salsa

2 cup diced peppers, I used red, orange and yellow

1 cup diced onion, I used red onion

1 cup reduced fat shredded cheese, I use a 3 cheese blend

Green onion

Fat free sour cream for topping, optional

Instructions:

Cook your ground beef in a pan on the stove, add your taco seasoning and simmer for a few minutes.

Preheat oven to 350F, spray a 9x13 casserole dish and set aside.

Mix your ground beef and salsa together in a bowl.

Cut up peppers & onion, and cut your biscuits into 6 pieces each.

Place half of your biscuit pieces in the bottom of your casserole dish, top with half of your meat mixture, half of your peppers and onions and half of your cheese. Repeat layers and finish with your chopped green onion on top.

Loosely cover with foil and bake in oven for 35 minutes, remove foil and continue baking for 15 minutes.Let cool for 5 minutes then cut into 6 servings. 7sp or 6pp per serving. Top with a spoon of fat free sour cream (optional)

Tater Tot Casserole

Ingredients:

23 oz Ore-Ida Tater Tots

2 can canned condensed cream of mushroom / chicken soup

4 oz low-fat cheddar or colby cheese

1 pound Morningstar Farms Frozen Burger Style Recipe Crumbles

1 onion, chopped

Green beans, mixed veggies, your choice

Instructions:

1. Preheat oven to 350. Sautee onions in pan sprayed with Pam. Add veggies, then veggie crumbles. Stir until heated through. Mix onion mixture with soups (don't add water.)

2. Spray 9x13 pan with Pam. Place onion mixture in bottom of pan. Put cheese over the mix. Layer tater tots on top.

3. Bake 30 to 45 minutes until tater tots are golden brown and mixture is bubbly hot.

Creamy Pasta salad

Ingredients:

8oz whole wheat pasta

2 medium cucumbers, diced

1 red bell pepper, diced

1 cup broccoli, chopped

1 small red onion, diced

1 3-4oz can sliced black olives,drained

1/2 cup plain, non-fat Greek yogurt

1/4 cup reduced fat mayonnaise (I used Vegenaise)

1 tbsp sugar

2 tbsp white vinegar

Salt & pepper to taste

Instructions:

Cook pasta according to package directions. Right before removing the pasta from the heat, add broccoli to the water, and cook for about 45 seconds. Drain pasta and broccoli, and rinse well with cold water.

Place pasta and broccoli in a large bowl and add in bell pepper, onions, cucumber and black olives. Toss to combine.

In a small bowl, whisk together the yogurt, mayo, sugar, vinegar and salt & pepper. Pour over pasta salad and toss well to coat. Cover and refrigerate until ready to serve.

Preparation time: 15 minute(s)

Cooking time: 15 minute(s)

Diet type: Vegetarian.

Pineapple food cake

Ingredients:

1 box (1-step) angel food cake mix (I used Betty Crocker)

1 large can (about 20 ounces) crushed pineapple, undrained

Instructions:

Preheat oven to 350F degrees.

In a large bowl, stir together the dry cake and the entire can of crushed pineapple with its juice. Stir well until all the dry mix is incorporated. (The mixture will get really foamy.)

Pour the batter into a 9x13 pan which has been lightly greased with nonstick cooking spray.

Bake at 350F degrees for time specified on the box for size pan. When the sides pull away from pan and toothpick inserted in the center comes out clean, the cake is done. This should take somewhere between 30 and 40 minutes.

Remove from the oven and place on a wire rack to cool.

Chapter 15 : 8 Points recipes

No-bake peanut butter cheerio bars

Ingredients:

1 cup of peanut butter

2 tsp of vanilla extract

1 cup of peanuts

5 cups of Cheerios cereal or peanut butte r Cheerios

1/2 cup of white sugar

1/2 cup of corn syrup

1 scoop of vanilla protein powder(optional)

2 tablespoons of mini chocolate chips (optional)

Instructions:

In a medium saucepan mix together white sugar and light corn syrup. Bring to a boil. Add peanut butter, vanilla and protein powder. Mix until smooth.

Place peanut butter Cheerios and peanuts in a large mixing bowl. Pour peanut butter mixture over Cheerios and peanuts. Stir until combined.

Spread Cheerio mixture in a 9 x 13 inch pan that has been greased with non-stick cooking spray.

Easy Taco Salad

Ingredients:

12 ounces ground round

2 cups chopped yellow, red, or green bell pepper

2 cups bottled salsa

1/4 cup chopped fresh cilantro

4 cups coarsely chopped romaine lettuce

2 cups chopped plum tomato

1 cup (4 ounces) shredded reduced-fat sharp cheddar cheese

1 cup crumbled baked tortilla chips (about 12 chips)

1/4 cup chopped green onions.

Directions:

Cook beef and bell pepper in a large nonstick skillet over medium-high heat until beef is browned; stir to crumble. Add salsa; bring to a boil. Stir in cilantro; keep warm.

Place 1 cup lettuce on each of 4 plates; top with 1 cup meat mixture. Sprinkle each serving with 1/2 cup tomato, 1/4 cup cheese, 1/4 cup chips, and 1 tablespoon onions.

Makes 4 Equal Servings

Nutrition Information:

Calories 330, Cholesterol 68 mg, Fat 11 g, Carbs 28 g, Fiber 6 g, Protein 32 g.

Chicken baked ziti

Ingredients:

2 tablespoons of all purpose flour

2 tablespoons of light butter

6 oz of fat free cream cheese

1/4 cup of Franks Original Buffalo Wing Sauce

1 tablespoon of ranch seasoning

4 oz of Rotisserie Chicken

5 cups of ziti noodles (or penne)

2 cups of fat free milk

chives for garnish

1/2 cup of low fat colby jack cheese

Instructions:

Preheat oven to 350 degrees F. In a large pot of salted boiling water, cook pasta until al dente. Drain and return to pot.

Make sauce: In a large skillet over medium heat, melt butter. Add flour and whisk to combine. Cook 1 minute. Add milk and whisk until combined and no clumps remain. Simmer until thickened, 2 minutes. Add cream cheese and break up with a wooden spoon until melted and combined. Add Frank's and ranch seasoning and stir until combined.

Add chicken, chives, and cooked ziti to skillet and stir until pasta is completely coated. Top with a layer of colby jack cheese and bake until melted and golden, 15 minutes.

Garnish with chives and serve.

Chicken Enchiladas

Ingredients:

2 large chicken breast filets with skin (remove skin before adding to enchiladas)

1 (16 ounce) jar red enchilada sauce (no sugar added)

1 (4 ounce) can jalapenos, optional green chiles

1/2 teaspoon garlic powder

1 teaspoon cumin

1 teaspoon chili powder

1/2 teaspoon black pepper

1 1/2 cups shredded cheddar cheese, reduced fat

1 (8 oz.) container sour cream, fat free

6 medium whole grain tortillas, (corn tortillas are not recommended as they tend to fall apart)

Instructions:

Preheat oven to 350 degrees. Place chicken breasts in a covered baking dish. Bake until juices run clear when pierced with a fork, after about 35-45 minutes. Remove skin and discard. Shred chicken or cut into bite-sized cubes.

In a medium mixing bowl add chicken, garlic powder, cumin, chili powder, black pepper, and salt to taste. Add to seasoned chicken: green chile peppers, 1/2 cup of enchilada sauce, 1/2 cup sour cream, and 1 cup cheese. Mix well. Place 1/2 cup chicken mixture in the center of each tortilla. Leave about 2" in the bottom without filling and fold up. Continue until all tortillas are filled.

Stack enchiladas in the slow cooker, add a little of the sauce on top of each layer as you stack them. There should be 2 layers of 3 or 3 layers of 2, depending on the size of your slow cooker.

Combine the remaining enchilada sauce and 1/2 cup sour cream. Pour over the enchiladas. Cover and cook on low 3 to 4 hours, or until hot and bubbly. Cut between each enchilada, and carefully remove them, one at a time, with a large spatula. Pour liquid from slow cooker over enchiladas and sprinkle with remaining cheese. Garnish with diced tomatoes and shredded lettuce.

Sheet pan Italian chicken and veggie dinner

Ingredients:

FOR THE SEASONING:

1 teaspoon kosher salt

1/2 teaspoon onion powder

1/2 teaspoon dried oregano

1/2 teaspoon dried basil

1/4 teaspoon thyme

1/2 teaspoon sugar (omit for Paleo and Whole 30)

1/8 teaspoon black pepper

1 clove crushed garlic

3 tablespoons olive oil

2 tablespoons red wine vinegar

FOR THE SHEETPAN:

cooking spray

8 (4 oz each) boneless skinless chicken thighs, trimmed of fat

1/2 tsp kosher salt

12 ounces zucchini, diced into 1-inch pieces

3 carrots, peeled and diced into 1-inch pieces

1 red bell pepper, cut into 1-inch pieces

1 yellow bell pepper, cut into 1-inch pieces

1 red onion, cut into 1-inch pieces

chopped parsley for garnish

Directions:

Preheat oven to 450F degrees. Spray 2 large nonstick sheetpans with oil or use parchment or foil for easy cleanup. Arrange the center rack and lower third.

Combine the Italian seasoning ingredients in a large bowl. Season chicken with 1/2 teaspoon salt, then add the chicken, zucchini, carrots, bell peppers and red onion to the bowl and toss well to coat. Marinate 30 minutes or as long as overnight.

Arrange everything onto the prepared baking sheets spread out into a single layer. The vegetables and chicken should not touch. Bake about 20 minutes, turn chicken and vegetables and bake an additional 10 minutes, until roasted and tender. Top with fresh parsley and serve

Hawaiian Chicken

Ingredients:

4-6 boneless, skinless chicken breasts

1 can (8 oz.) crushed pineapple, drained

1 bottle (16 ounces) barbeque sauce

Instructions:

Place chicken in a greased 3.5-5 quart crock pot

Combine drained pineapple and BBQ sauce in a bowl and pour over meat

Cook on high heat for 3-4 hours or on low heat for 6-8 hours

Serve over rice.

Layered Chicken Enchilada Bake

Ingredients:

2 (10 oz) cans red enchilada sauce, divided

9 (6 inch) yellow corn tortillas

1 (16 oz) can fat free refried beans

4 teaspoons canola oil

1 ½ lbs boneless, skinless chicken breasts, chopped into small bite-sized pieces (about ½")

1 medium onion, diced

1 cup drained and rinsed canned black beans

¾ cup frozen corn kernels

6 oz 50% light sharp cheddar cheese, shredded

Directions:

Pre-heat the oven to 350. Lightly mist a 9×13 baking dish with cooking spray. Drizzle about 1/3 cup of the enchilada sauce across the bottom of the dish and spread around with the back of a spoon to lightly coat the bottom of the dish. Arrange 4 ½ of the tortillas across the bottom of the dish to cover the majority of the space (my arrangement is pictured above). Use a spatula to spread the refried beans evenly across the tortillas, forming an even layer across the whole dish. Set aside.

In a large skillet or saute pan, bring the oil to medium heat. Add the chopped chicken and diced onion and stir to coat in the oil.

Cook, stirring occasionally, until the chicken is cooked through and the onions are softened (6-10 minutes). Drain the liquid from the pan if necessary. Add all the remaining enchilada sauce, the black beans and the corn and stir together. Remove from heat.

Spoon about half of the chicken and sauce mixture evenly across the top of the refried bean layer in the casserole dish. Sprinkle about half of the cheddar cheese evenly across as well. Arrange the remaining 4 ½ tortillas in a similar style to step 1 (I did the same but flipped the layout so any small missing spots from layer 1 would be covered and vice versa). Spoon the remaining chicken and sauce mixture evenly across the newly laid tortillas. Sprinkle the remaining cheese over the top. Bake in the oven for 30 minutes. Cut into 8 pieces and serve.

Skinny Cheeseburger Stuffed Peppers.

Ingredients:

1 cup cooked brown rice

1 pound extra lean ground beef (96%), see shopping tip

1 cup onions, diced

Salt and pepper, to taste

2 tablespoons Worcestershire sauce (for gluten-free use Lea & Perrins)

2 tablespoons ketchup

1 tablespoon mustard (I used a spicy brown mustard)

1 tablespoon pickle relish

? cup tomato sauce, can or jarred

3 tablespoons water

1 cup lite cheddar cheese, mozzarella or blend, shredded (I used Trader's lite Mexican blend)

4 large red bell peppers, yellow or orange (each about 3½ inches high and 3½ inches wide)

Instructions:

1. Cook rice and set aside. Cut off the top of 4 bell peppers about 1-inch down from top. Clean out seeds and membranes. Throw away the tops.

2. Preheat oven to 400 degrees.

3. In a large nonstick pan, brown ground beef and onions. Season beef with a little salt and pepper. Be sure to break up ground beef into small pieces as it cooks.

4. Stir in Worcestershire sauce, ketchup, mustard, pickle relish, tomato sauce and 3 tablespoons water. Mix well. Stir in ¾ cup shredded cheese and cooked rice. Mix well and continue to cook until heated through. Add 1-2 more tablespoons of water, if getting a little dry. Remove from heat.

5. Stuff each bell pepper with ground beef mixture, top each stuffed pepper with 1 tablespoon shredded cheese. Place each in a 9-inch baking dish. Pour 1 cup water in bottom of baking dish. Cover dish with foil and bake for 40-45 minutes. If peppers are not soft enough, cook about 5 minutes more.

6. Once cooked, cooled and wrapped, they freeze great!

Makes 4 servings. Each serving, 1 stuffed pepper.

Shopping Tip

Happily most supermarkets sell extra lean ground beef. I used the 96% lean ground beef from Trader Joe's. You could use ground turkey, if desired.

Sloppy JOE'S

Ingredients:

1 pound extra lean (95%) ground beef

3/4 cup Picante Sauce

1/2 cup barbecue sauce

2 green onions, sliced (about 1/4 cup, optional)

5 light hamburger buns, split and lightly toasted

Instructions:

In a large skillet set over medium high heat, cook the beef, stirring and breaking up the meat, until it is browned, 5 to 10 minutes.

Add the picante sauce, barbecue sauce and green onions (if using) into the skillet. Stir to combine.

Cook, stirring often, until the mixture is hot and bubbling.

Divide the beef mixture evenly among the five buns.

Chapter 16 : 9 Points recipes

Grilled Chicken Skewers with Peanut Sauce

Ingredients:

1 1/2 pounds chicken breast fillets (about 4 fillets) cut lengthwise into 12 strips

1/2 cup lite soy sauce, optional Tamari

2 tablespoons sesame oil

2 tablespoons honey

1 teaspoon balsamic vinegar

2 cloves garlic, minced

2 teaspoons freshly grated ginger

2 teaspoons red pepper flakes

Peanut Sauce

1/2 cup natural peanut butter, creamy or crunchy

1 tablespoon honey

2 tablespoons lite soy sauce, optional Tamari

2 teaspoons freshly grated ginger

2 tablespoons freshly squeezed lime juice

1 clove garlic, minced

1/2 teaspoon red pepper flakes

1/4 cup water

12 small (6 inch) skewers

Instructions:

Whisk together soy sauce, sesame oil, honey, vinegar, garlic, minced ginger, and red pepper flakes. Place chicken strips in marinade, cover, refrigerate, and let sit overnight or at least 5 hours.

Peanut Sauce: Add all ingredients to a food processor or blender and pluse until smooth. Add additional water if a thinner consistency is desired. Pour sauce into a glass dish or jar, cover and refrigerate until ready to serve.

Thread skewers with marinated chicken strips and refrigerate while heating the remaining marinate. Pour the remaining marinate into a small sauce pan, bring to a boil, reduce heat and simmer until thickened.

Lightly oil grates of grill, grill pan, or skillet with canola or coconut oil, and turn to medium-high heat. Once hot, add skewers and cook for about 3-4 minutes per side, or until chicken is cooked through and lightly browned, basting with the marinade as it cooks.

Serve Chicken Skewers with Peanut Sauce. Enjoy!

Baked Cream cheese spaghetti casserole

Ingredients:

12 oz spaghetti

1 (28 ounce) jars prepared spaghetti sauce

1 lb lean ground beef lean ground turkey

1 tsp Italian seasoning

1 clove garlic, minced

8 ounces cream cheese fat free cream cheese

1/2 cup parmesan cheese, grated

Instructions:

Preheat oven to 350 F degrees.

In a skillet, brown the ground beef until cooked through; drain fat and stir in spaghetti sauce. Set aside.

Cook spaghetti according to directions on packet. Drain and place cooked spaghetti in bowl. Add cream cheese, Italian Seasoning and minced garlic. Stir until cream cheese is melted and the spaghetti is thoroughly coated.

Turkey Chili Mac with Jalapeños

Ingredients:

1 teaspoon granulated garlic

1 teaspoon onion powder

1 teaspoon ground coriander

1 teaspoon cumin

2 teaspoons chili power

¼ salt, plus more to taste if needed

1 tablespoon olive oil

1 lb ground turkey

3 cups beef broth

1 (10-ounce) can diced tomatoes with green chilis

2 cups dry whole wheat elbow pasta

½ cup pickled jalapenos, chopped

½ cup 1% milk

4 ounces cream cheese

1 cup shredded sharp cheddar cheese

Instructions:

In a small bowl mix together granulated garlic, onion powder, ground coriander, cumin, chili powder and salt.

In a large pot or Dutch oven heat olive oil on medium high. Add ground turkey and cook until no longer pink. Stir in the spices and cook for another 1-2 minutes.

Stir in beef broth, diced tomatoes, and dry pasta. Cook for about 8-10 minutes or until the pasta is cooked.

While the pasta is cooking pour milk into a small pot and heat up slowly over low heat. After the milk is warm and steaming add the cream cheese and stir until it is melted.

Add the shredded cheese to the milk and cream cheese. Stir until it is melted.

Pour the cheese sauce into the pasta mixture and stir until the pasta is evenly coated.

Stir in the pickled jalapenos. Give it a taste and add a little more salt if needed. Serve hot.

Crock Pot Teriyaki Chicken

Ingredients Serves 6:

2 1/2 lb boneless, skinless chicken breast, cut into 2 inch pieces

1/2 cup soy sauce

1/2 cup honey

3 whole garlic cloves

1 hot chili sauce, optional

Directions:

Prep 5 min Cook 240 min Ready 245 min

Add chicken to a crock pot with soy sauce, honey, garlic cloves and hot chili sauce, if using.

Set the crock pot to Low and cover.

Stir after 2 hours and then cook an additional 2 hours.

Remove garlic cloves.

Beef tips

Ingredients :

1 small onion, sliced

8 oz baby Bella mushrooms, sliced

1 tbsp extra virgin olive oil

1 lb sirloin steak, cut in strips, excess fat trimmed

Salt & pepper

1 tbsp Worcestershire sauce

¼ cup dry red wine + splash for deglazing

2-½ cups fat free beef broth

2 tbsp corn starch + ¼ cup cold water, whisked together.

Preparation :

Place the onions and mushrooms into the bottom of a 4.5 quart slow cooker.

Then, heat the oil in a large skillet over medium-high heat. Generously season the steak strips with salt and pepper and add them to the hot skillet, and sear the meat on all sides, about 3 minutes; do not cook through.

Place the meat into the slow cooker on top of the vegetables.

Splash a couple tablespoons of red wine into the hot skillet and scrape the bottom to remove any browned meat bits. Add these to the crock pot.

Season the beef with pepper a second time and add the Worcestershire sauce, red wine, and beef broth. Cover and cook on low for 6-8 hours.

Uncover and slowly whisk in the cornstarch and water mixture. Cover and cook on high for another 45 minutes or until the gravy has thickened.

Serve the beef tips over brown rice (shown), buttered egg noodles, or mashed potatoes.

Chapter 17 : 10 Points recipes

Deli crab salad

Ingredients:

6 ounces imitation crab meat

2 tablespoons light mayo

Chopped green onion or chives

1/2 to 1 teaspoon mustard

1/4 cup fat free sour cream

onion powder (to taste)

salt and pepper (to taste)

1 cup cooked macaroni noodles

Instructions:

Cook noodles and measure out 1 cup. Run cold water over the noodles to chill them. Mix the shredded or diced crab pieces with the pasta. Mix in green onions or chives. In a separate bowl, mix remaining ingredients. Pour sauce over pasta mixture and stir well. Put it in the fridge for a few hours or overnight to let the flavors blend.

Bubble up pizza

Ingredients:

1 pound 96% lean ground beef

2 teaspoons onion powder, or 1 onion, chopped

16 ounces tomato sauce

1/2 teaspoon dried basil

3 cloves garlic, minced

1 teaspoon Italian seasoning

15 ounces refrigerated buttermilk biscuits, buttermilk

Add whatever typical pizza toppings you like, green pepper, turkey pepperoni, mushrooms, etc.

1 1/4 cups part skim milk mozzarella cheese, shredded

Instructions:

Preheat oven to 350 F. In skillet, brown meat over medium high heat until browned, stirring to crumble. Stir in onion powder, tomato sauce, basil, garlic and Italian seasoning.

Add quartered biscuits; stir gently until biscuits are covered with sauce. Mix in toppings of your choosing. Spoon mixture into a 9×13 inch baking dish coated with cooking spray. Bake for 25 minutes. Sprinkle with cheese; bake an additional 10 minutes or until biscuits are done. Let stand 5 minutes before serving.

Chicken Cacciatore with Pasta

Ingredients Serves 4:

1 lb (four 4 oz pieces) boneless, skinless chicken breast, pounded thin

1/2 tsp salt

1/4 tsp black pepper

1 tsp olive oil

1 medium onion, chopped

1 medium green pepper, chopped

1 medium yellow pepper, chopped

1 clove garlic, minced

1/2 cup beef broth or dry red wine

1 can (29 oz) italian style stewed tomatoes

2 tbsp fresh parsley, chopped

3 cup cooked linguine or spaghetti

Directions:

Prep 15 min Cook 30 min Ready 45 min

Season chicken with salt and pepper. Heat olive oil in a large nonstick skillet over medium heat. Add chicken breasts and cook until browned, about 5 minutes on each side. Add onion, peppers, and garlic to the skillet and cook until the vegetables have softened. Stir in beef broth or red wine and tomatoes. Bring to boil, reduce heat to medium-low, cover, and simmer for 20 minutes. Sprinkle with parsley and serve with pasta.

Buffalo Chicken Lasagna

Ingredients:

Main Ingredients

Whole wheat lasagna noodles (uncooked)12

Skinless chicken breast (cooked and cubed)1 lb.

Water1½ cups

Non-fat ricotta cheese15 oz.

Egg substitute½ cup

Pepper jack cheese½ cup

Seasoning

Spaghetti sauce3 cups

Texas Pete Buffalo-style wing sauce1 cup

Instructions:

1. Preheat the oven till it reaches 350 degrees.

2. Combine egg substitute and ricotta cheese in a small mixing bowl then set it aside.

3. Combine chicken, wing sauce, water and spaghetti sauce in another mixing bowl.

4. Spread about a cup of the mixture of chicken and sauce on a baking pan and place in four noodles on top of the sauce.

5. Spread over the noodles a layer of sauce followed by a layer of the ricotta cheese mixture.

6. Add some more noodles in just the same way, then sauce, ricotta cheese mixture and finally a layer of sauce and chicken mixture.

7. Cover the pan with aluminum foil then let it bake for an hour.

8. Remove the dish, sprinkle pepper jack cheese on top and again bake for 15 minutes uncovered.

Granola with Raisins

Ingredients Serves 12:

4 cup old fashioned oats

1/2 cup sliced almond

1/2 cup light brown sugar, packed

1/2 tsp salt

1/2 tsp cinnamon

1/4 cup cooking oil

1/4 cup honey

1 tsp vanilla

1 1/2 cup raisins or dried cranberry

Directions:

Prep 10 min Cook 40 min Ready 50 min

In a bowl, mix oats, almonds, brown sugar, salt and cinnamon. In a sauce pan, warm the oil and honey. Whisk or stir in the vanilla. Carefully pour liquid over the oat mixture. Stir gently with wooden spoon, finish mixing by hand.

Preheat oven to 300°F Spread granola in a 15x10x1" pan. Bake 40 minutes, stirring carefully every 10 minutes.

Transfer granola-filled pan to a cooling rack. Cool completely.

Stir in raisins or dried cranberries. Seal granola in an air-tight container or self sealing plastic bags.

Store at room temperature for 1 week or the freezer for 3 months.

Skinny Berry Parfait

Ingredients:

1 cup old-fashioned oats

1/2 cup almonds with skins, sliced

1/2 teaspoon cinnamon

3 tablespoons unrefined coconut oil

1/2 cup fresh raspberries

1/2 cup fresh blueberries

1/2 cup fresh blackberries

2 cups raspberry yogurt (here's the recipe, just change out strawberry spread for raspberry)

Instructions:

Preheat oven to 350 degrees.

In a medium bowl, combine oats, almonds and cinnamon. Stir in melted coconut oil to combine with other ingredients. Line a cookie sheet with parchment, spread oats evenly and bake approximately 20 minutes or until golden. Stir after 10 minutes. Allow to cool completely.

You'll likely have leftover granola. This granola is a wonderful snack or topping. Try adding rasins or other dried fruit without added sweeteners.

Alternate yogurt, granola and berries in parfait glasses.

Choose other berries if you prefer.

Syn Free And Sour Chicken

Ingredients:

10 Chicken Thighs skin removed

1 large Onion chopped

1 tbsp Garlic minced

1 tsp Chilli optional - we like it in ours

1 tbsp Ginger chopped finely

5 Mushrooms quartered

1 large Celery stick chopped

1 large Carrots chopped

125 ml Water

2 Chicken Stock Cubes

1 large Yellow Bell Pepper sliced

1 large Red Bell Pepper sliced

1 large Green Bell Pepper sliced

1 bunch spring onions chopped

4 tbsp Soy Sauce

2 tbsp Rice Vinegar

2 tbsp fish sauce

2 tbsp Lemon Juice

2 tbsp Sweetener

4 tbsp Tomato Puree

1/2 tsp Xanthan Gum

1/2 Fresh Pineapple cut into chunks

Instructions:

Slow Cooker Method

Remove the skin from the thighs & season well. Mist a pan with Frylight and heat

In a jug - add the soy sauce, rice vinegar, fish sauce, lemon juice, sweetener & tomato puree, water and 2 chicken stock cubes and mix well. Set aside.

Brown the chicken thighs in small batches in the pan, then keep them to one side

Deglaze the pan with some of the water, and make sure to scrape the bits of chicken off the bottom if any had stuck, pour this into your slow cooker

Add the chopped onions, carrots, celery, mushrooms, chilli, garlic and ginger to the slow cooker & layer the browned chicken thighs on top. Pour the jug of sauce over the chicken

Place the lid on the slow cooker & cook on High for 4-5 hours

At 4 hours in - remove the chicken thighs and set aside. In a jug measure out the xanthan gum and add a few tablespoons of the sauce in the slow cooker. Mix well until the lumps are gone and it's turned into a paste. Add this to the sauce in the pot.

Add the chicken back into the pot, along with the peppers and spring onion. LEAVING THE LID OFF cook for a further 30-60 minutes

Turn the slow cooker off and stir the pineapple through. Serve immediately.

Mushroom and Steak Fajita Sandwiches

Ingredients:

1 tablespoon plus 2 teaspoons olive oil

1 medium red onion, sliced in to strips

2 cloves garlic, minced

1 medium red bell pepper, cut into strips

1 pound beef sirloin tip steak, cut into thin strips (grass-fed beef recommended)

4 ounces white mushrooms, sliced

2 teaspoons dried oregano

1/2 teaspoon black pepper

Salt to taste

2 whole wheat pita pockets cut in half

4 leaves of Romaine lettuce, torn into small pieces

1/4 cup Greek yogurt, fat free, plain (optional fat free sour cream)

Instructions:

Preheat oven to 350 degrees.

In a large skillet, on medium-low heat, sauté mushrooms in 1 tablespoon olive oil, about 6 minutes. Add onions, garlic and bell peppers and continue sautéing until onions and peppers are tender, about 4 minutes minutes. Add in sirloin strips, and cook on medium heat for about 5-10 minutes or until no longer pink. Sprinkle with salt and pepper and oregano. Stir well, cover and simmer for 5 more minutes. Drain mixture.

Cut pita bread in half, brush remaining oil on all sides, place on a cookie sheet for 3-5 minutes, just long enough to warm. Stuff pita pockets with meat mixture, romaine lettuce and top with a dollop of yogurt or sour cream.

Conclusion

This diet can be followed only for a short period of time, in order not to face health problems. It is also useful to reaffirm that it is always essential to have a proper diet prescribed by your nutritionist or dietician.

What the points diet promises, is the loss of about 3-4 kg per month, especially in the abdominal area.

The positive aspects of this diet are that it is a relatively easy diet to follow. In fact, it presents a few simple rules and it is not necessary to calculate the calories that are ingested obsessively. It allows you to eat the right and in a healthy way.

Basically, it is an interesting diet, to be tried especially for those who want to lose fat located in a specific part of the body.